Stress Remedy

Dr. Sheila Harrison

Disclaimer

This content serves to provide general information about the disease and aims to empower you to seek prompt medical assistance if necessary to prevent complications. It's essential to stress that this information is not a substitute for consulting a qualified physician. The field of medical science is continually evolving, and due to the dynamic nature of medical knowledge, we recommend seeking expert advice if you encounter any inconsistencies or intend to take action based on the information in this content. Never disregard professional medical guidance or delay treatment based on something you've read online, including this material, or from any other online source. Always remember that the internet cannot cure you; rather, healing comes through the guidance of medical professionals and the providence of God.

Table of Content

Section 1

Mind and Health

(How our Mindset Plays a massive role in resisting stress)

Have you ever pondered how the body handles stress? The brain creates its own cannabinoid molecules to help us relax during stressful situations. These molecules activate the same brain receptors as Tetrahydrocannabinol (THC), which is generated from cannabis plants. This has been discovered by researchers, including one of Indian descent. However, little was known about the neural circuits and patterns of brain activity that these cannabinoid molecules derived from the brain regulate.

Stress increases the likelihood that mental illnesses such as major depressive disorder, post-traumatic stress disorder (PTSD), and generalized anxiety disorder will manifest or worsen. Comprehending the molecular, cellular, and circuit mechanisms by which the brain adjusts to stress may offer crucial understanding of the ways in which stress manifests as mood disorders and may also identify new therapeutic targets for the management of stress-related conditions.

Modern Western medicine has mostly focused on using medications and surgery to alter the body's mechanical systems. Psychosocial variables, however, have a significant impact on who becomes unwell, how long they stay sick, and how well they recover. The key is stress, or perhaps more properly, our feelings of stress.

pain in the chest, back, headache, dizziness, breathing problems, insomnia, pain in the abdomen, and low energy. Do you recognize this? These are the most typical causes for why people see a doctor.

Even after a comprehensive patient history, physical examination, and medical testing, less than half of all patients exhibiting these symptoms receive an accurate diagnosis from their doctors, despite the fact that these conditions are quite frequent. Due to their failure to recognize psychological stress, which is the source of many physical symptoms and a prevalent root cause of human misery, doctors either fail to diagnose patients or do so incorrectly.

Stress Matters

Most patients experience what is best described as "everyday psychological distress," but 10 to 20 percent of them show severe anxiety and depression suggestive of a significant psychiatric disease. This more prevalent kind of psychological distress significantly affects daily social and physical functioning. It even results in impairments comparable to those caused by arthritis, diabetes, or hypertension.

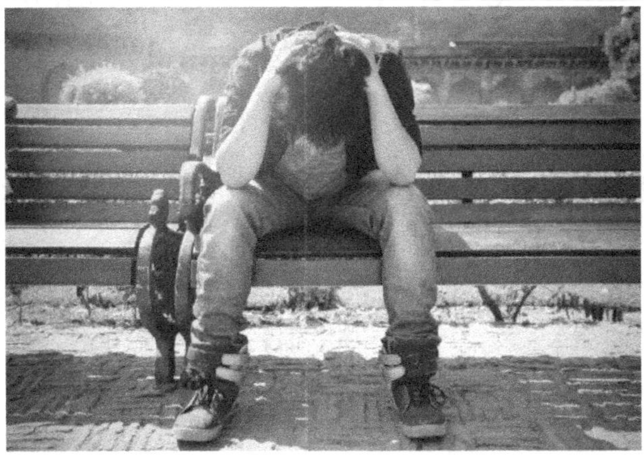

Unhealthy stress levels are reported by most Americans. Furthermore, 1 in 5 respondents describe their level of stress as "very high." Perhaps even more concerning is the fact that only 37% of Americans believe they can effectively control their stress. The most prevalent sources of stress include relationships, employment, family obligations, financial strains, and personal health issues.

Ironically, stress has a detrimental effect on the elements of people's life that first give rise to it. For example, seventy percent of people who are under stress report medical symptoms, decreased productivity at work, and disturbances in their social and familial lives.

Adults who experience high levels of stress are also less likely to manage their alcohol intake, eat sensibly, exercise, or get enough sleep. These habits, which are frequently brought on by stress, increase the risk of developing depression, cardiovascular disease, and even cold susceptibility. Even our DNA can be impacted by stress, hastening the aging process. When compared to women under less stress, women under severe stress have a shortening of certain regions of their DNA, which is comparable to over ten years of faster aging.

We are aware that signs of stress have a negative impact on people's health. However, studies also highlight the disastrous effects stress has on the productivity of the American workforce and the healthcare system as a whole. One-third of American workers say they experience significant stress at work. Additionally, it is estimated that the stress of the job costs the American business $300 billion annually in lost productivity, employee turnover, absenteeism, and workplace accidents. In the meantime, employees who report high levels of stress incur health care costs that are almost fifty percent higher.

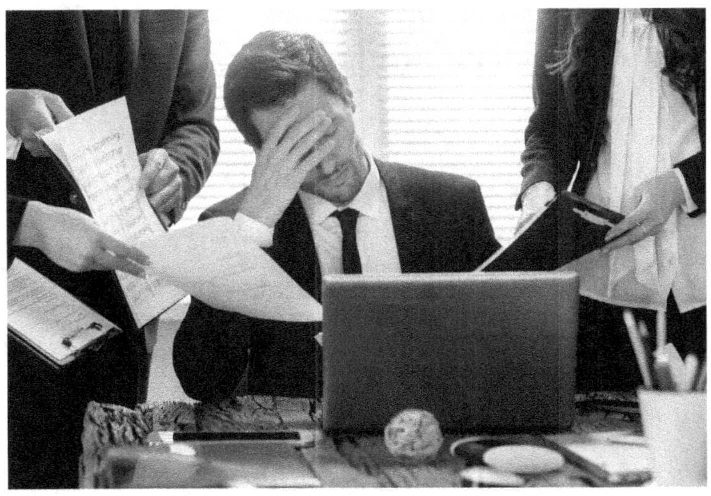

The Positive Side Of Stress: Positive Moods and Mindset Matters

Certain types of stress can be beneficial, especially if they spur required lifestyle adjustments and foster resilience. It's interesting to note that your perspective—or "mindset"—about the effects of stress on health and well-being appears to be moderating this effect. Individuals with a "stress-is-enhancing mindset," which sees stress as something that can be used and welcomed rather than something that should be avoided or decreased, fare considerably worse than those with a "stress-is-debilitating mindset."

Fortunately, it is possible to change these stress-related beliefs.

Research indicates that both happy and negative emotions have distinct effects on longevity and physical health. A growing body of research indicates that good biochemical and physiological consequences are attributed to happiness, pleasure, joy, optimism, excitement, and a sense of humor. Therefore, finding happiness is just as crucial to greater health as minimizing negativity and combating chronic stress.

Individuals who report being extremely happy—that is, having more positive and optimistic feelings and emotions—live between four and ten years longer than those who report being miserable. Furthermore, those extra years are spent in better health. In addition, those who exhibit happy, upbeat, and enthusiastic feelings had a 22% lower risk of heart disease than those who do not.

As a matter of fact, optimists had a 30% lower risk of dying from coronary heart disease than pessimists in a research involving almost 100,000 women. Happiness is a statistical predictor of health, even when it is expressed within a single day.

According to a study, people who felt happier within a 24-hour period had a 50% reduced death rate the next five years than people who felt less pleased on that day.

Given that happiness in all of its manifestations might enhance health, it begs the crucial question: Is it possible for us to choose happiness?

Can we change our general state of unhappiness, or are some people's emotional states impacted by their surroundings, upbringing, and genetics?

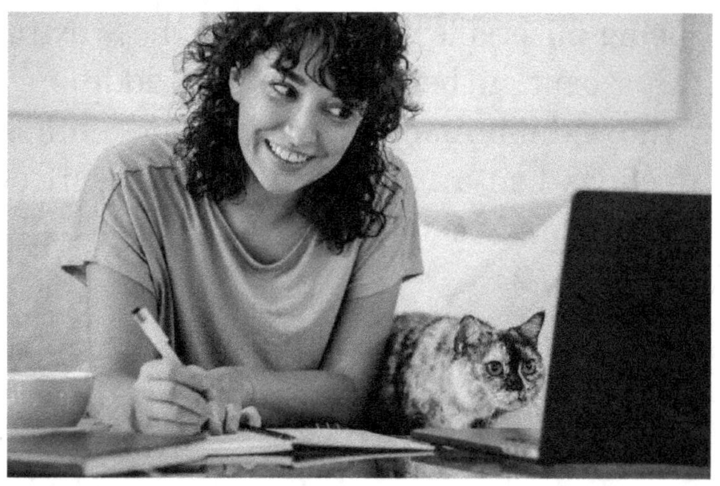

Of course, it's hard to pinpoint cause and effect in this case. Does negativity lead to stress, and stress has a detrimental effect on one's health? Can daily happiness also stop harmful health trends on its own? It is difficult to assess how stress levels affect changing one's lifestyle.

Disease prevalence and mood can be influenced by various factors, including genetics and environment. But whatever the cause, happy people handle such hardships better and maintain better health than miserable people.

Thankfully, there is growing proof that we can control our happiness and moods with a few easy practices and interventions that change our attitudes and ideas every day.

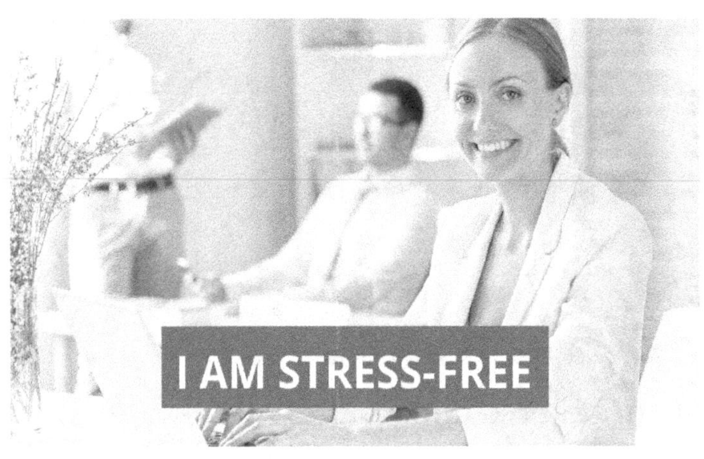

Section 2
What is Stress?

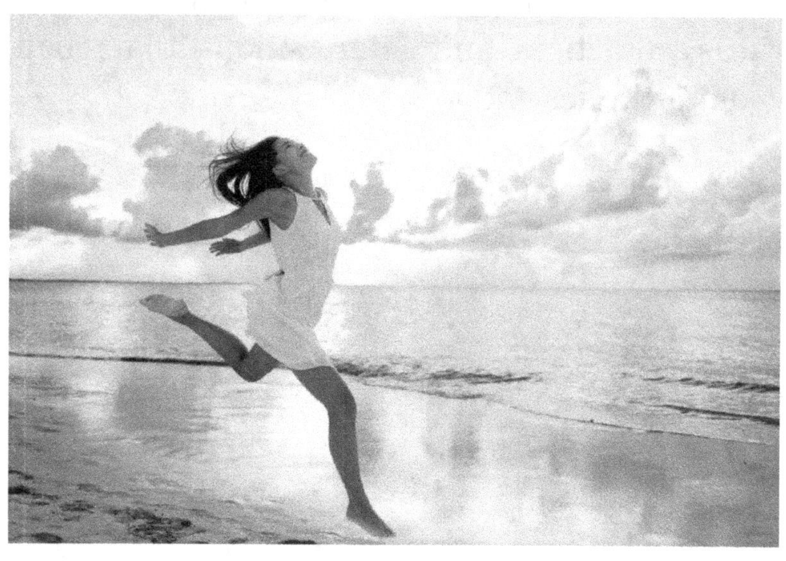

when you're under pressure or going through difficult events, you may have said, "I'm stressed," or "This is stressful." Although we may all relate to how it feels, what precisely is stress?

There are many advantages to comprehending stress and learning appropriate coping mechanisms. For example, effective stress management can spur someone to become more productive and finish all of their tasks on schedule.

Conversely, an inability to control stress can overwhelm a person and result in health issues

The way the body reacts to stress

Stress is a typical reaction of the body to changes, resulting in physical, emotional, and cognitive responses. Stress management training can assist you in dealing with changes in a more healthy manner.

It is critical to understand that stress is the body's normal reaction to external circumstances. They include academic, financial, health, relationship, and employment issues.

The autonomic nerve system of the body regulates your heart rate, respiration, visual changes, and other bodily functions. Its built-in stress response, known as the "fight-or-flight response," assists the body in dealing with stressful conditions.

When a person is under long-term (chronic) stress, the stress response is constantly activated, causing wear and tear on the body. Symptoms of physical, emotional, and behavioral nature emerge.

Symptoms of Stress

Physical symptoms of stress include:

- Aches and pains.
- Chest pain or a feeling like your heart is racing.
- Exhaustion or trouble sleeping.
- Headaches, dizziness or shaking.
- High blood pressure.
- Muscle tension or jaw clenching.
- Stomach or digestive problems.
- Trouble having sex.
- Weak immune system.

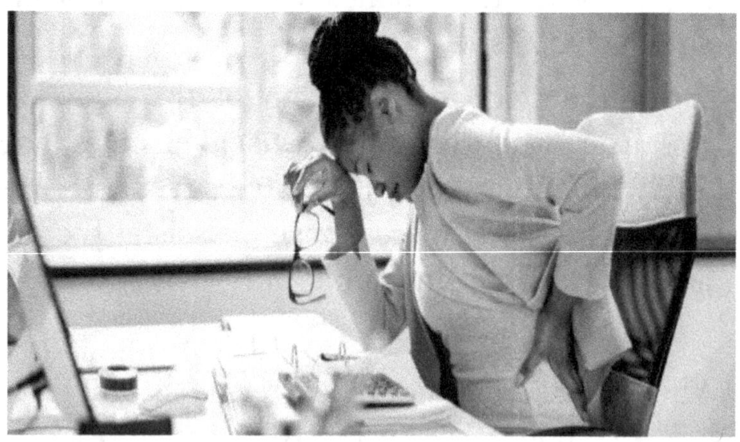

Stress can lead to emotional and mental symptoms like:

- Anxiety or irritability.
- Depression.
- Panic attacks.
- Sadness.

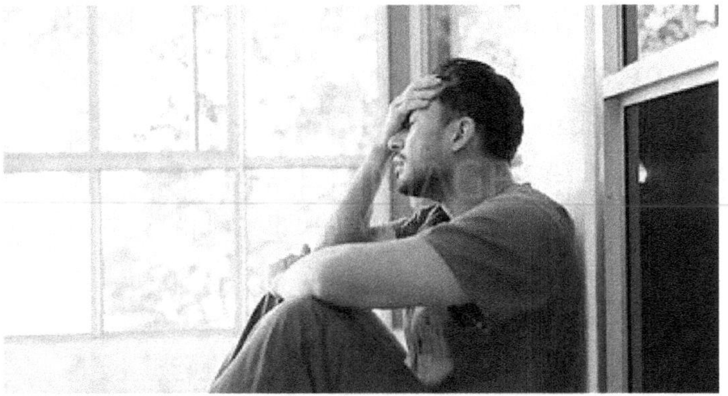

Often, people with chronic stress try to manage it with unhealthy behaviors, including:

- Drinking alcohol too much or too often.
- Gambling.
- Overeating or developing an eating disorder.
- Participating compulsively in sex, shopping or internet browsing.
- Smoking.
- Using drugs.

Diagnosis for Stress

Stress is not measured with testing because it is subjective. Only the individual experiencing it can tell if it is present and how terrible it is. Questionnaires may be used by a healthcare provider to better understand your stress and how it affects your life.

If you have chronic stress, your healthcare professional can assess stress-related symptoms. High blood pressure, for example, can be identified and treated.

Stress Relief Strategies

You cannot prevent stress, but you may keep it from becoming overwhelming by implementing the following everyday strategies:

- When you notice signs of stress, get some exercise. A brief walk might improve your mood.

- Take a minute at the end of each day to reflect on what you've accomplished rather than what you haven't.

- Set daily, weekly, and monthly objectives. Narrowing your focus will make you feel more in control of both short-term and long-term activities.

- Consider discussing your concerns with a therapist or your healthcare professional.

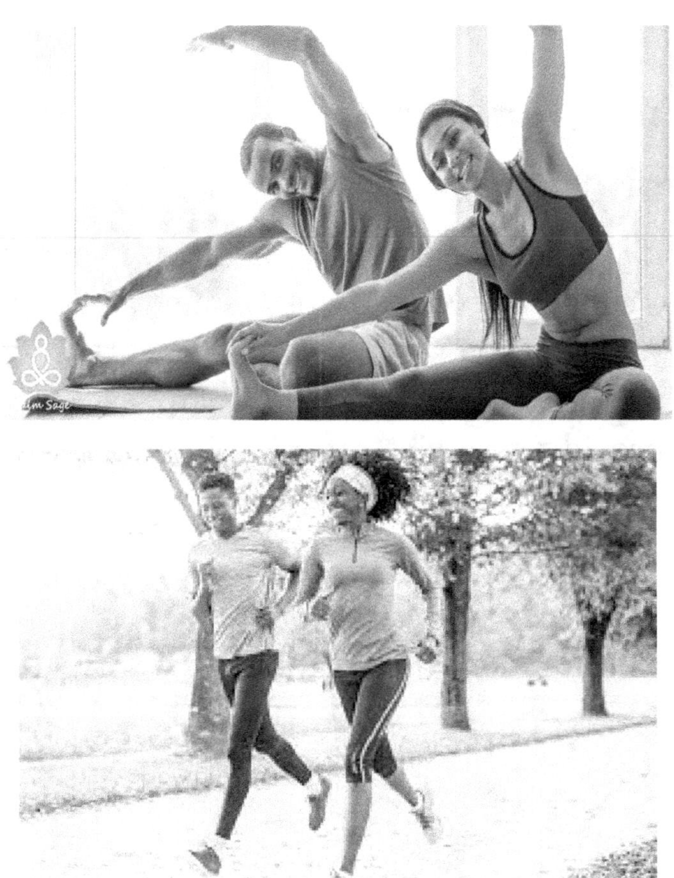

How long does stress last?

Depending on what happens in your life, stress can be a short-term or long-term problem. Most physical, mental, and behavioral effects of stress can be avoided by adopting stress management practices on a regular basis.

When should I talk to a doctor about stress?

If you are feeling overwhelmed, using drugs or alcohol to cope, or thinking about injuring yourself, you should get medical attention. Your primary care physician can assist you by providing advice, prescribing medication, or sending you to a therapist.

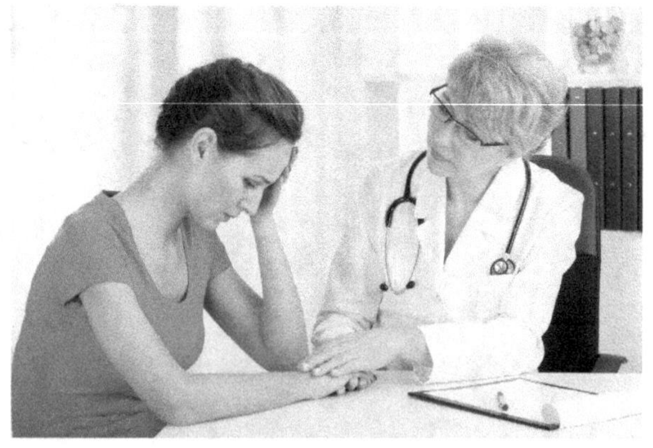

It's natural to feel worried from time to time. Long-term stress, on the other hand, can create medical symptoms, emotional problems, and undesirable habits. Try a few simple tactics for stress relief and management. However, if you are feeling overwhelmed, consult your doctor.

Stress Management

Although stress is expected in the current world's fast-paced lifestyle, it can be harmful when it occurs in the long term. Regular meditation can help calm your mind and muscles and reduce stress. Deep breathing can reduce the symptoms of stress. Social activity, sharing worries and some natural remedies can help relieve excess stress.

Stress is an indispensable aspect of modern life. Failure to address stress can have adverse effects on an individual's physical and mental health, overall well-being, and even socioeconomic status.

While stress, in moderation, can push you to perform better, excessive stress can be harmful to your body. To control stress in life, you can do the following:

- **Relaxation techniques:** Relaxation techniques such as deep breathing, meditation, yoga, Tai Chi, and progressive muscle relaxation can help reduce stress and promote relaxation. Try meditation for 30 minutes every day. You may find it difficult to concentrate initially, but with continuous practice, you will be able to see the difference in some time. Deep breathing counters the effect of stress by slowing down the heartbeat and lowering the blood pressure.

- **Exercise regularly:** Exercise is a great way to reduce stress, boost mood, and improve overall health. Aim for at least 30 minutes of physical activity most days of the week.

- **Improve your sleep cycle:** Getting enough restful sleep is important for overall health and well-being. Aim for 6-8 hours of sleep per night.

- **Socialize with people:** Talk to your friends or loved ones. Share your thoughts on what is keeping you stressed. Venting out, at times, helps.

- **Lifestyle changes:** Certain changes in lifestyle like reducing caffeine or alcohol intake and setting aside time for self-care and leisure activities may help as well.

- **Balanced diet:** The food we eat can affect our mood, energy levels, and overall health. A well-balanced diet can help provide the nutrients our bodies need to manage stress effectively.

- **Follow a daily routine:** It will help in utilizing time efficiently and feel more in control.

- Maintain a happy attitude and cultivate thankfulness, recognizing the positive aspects of your day or life.

- Recognize that you cannot control everything. Find strategies to let go of anxiety about things you can't control.

- When you are too busy or pressured, learn to say "no" to new tasks.

- Maintain contact with people who keep you calm, make you joyful, offer emotional support, and assist you with practical matters. So that tension does not become overpowering, a friend, family member, or neighbor can become a good listener or share tasks.

Also, it's important to note that what works for one person may not work for another and that it may take some trial and error to find the right combination of stress management techniques that work for you. Stress can have deleterious effects on health, such as depression, and erectile dysfunction. Remember, stress is not always bad. However, if it is becoming overwhelming and affecting your daily life, consider seeking professional help from a therapist or counselor.

Section 3

Handling Stress in Children from a Psychiatrist's Perspective

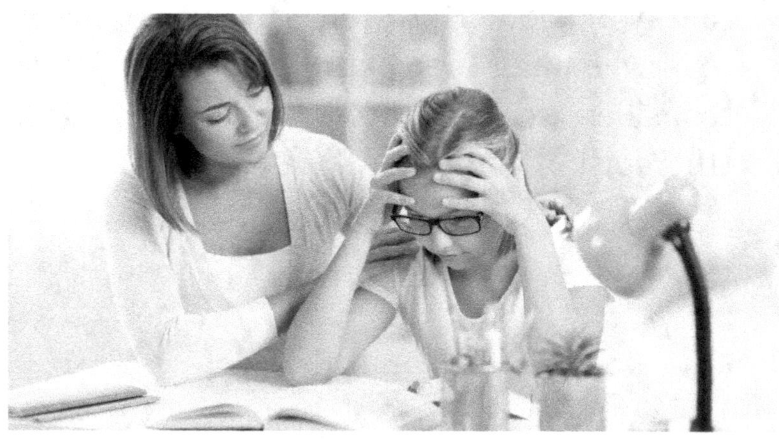

Children, like adults, can suffer stress. Expectations, peer pressure, and family issues are all examples of stressors.

Some stress in children can be beneficial, such as stress associated with beginning a new hobby or learning a new subject. However, too much of it might be harmful to a child.

Sometimes parents are unaware that their child is stressed. It is feasible, however, to learn about the signs and symptoms of stress in your children.

Early childhood stress appears to have a particularly profound effect throughout life. A long-term study of 17,000 adults discovered that negative childhood experiences are extremely common:

- 11% were subjected to emotional abuse.
- 28% were subjected to physical abuse.
- 21% had been sexually abused.
- 15% were subjected to emotional neglect.
- 10% were subjected to physical abuse.
- 13% witnessed their mothers being violently treated.
- 27% grew up in a home where someone used alcohol or drugs.
- 19% grew up in a household with a mentally ill person, and 23% lost a parent due to separation or divorce.
- 5% grew up with a family member who was in jail or prison.

The study also discovered that these youngsters have long-term, negative consequences. The more types of childhood trauma encountered, the more likely it is to experience:

- alcoholism and alcohol abuse
- COPD (chronic obstructive pulmonary disease)
- Ischemia (heart illness)
- Obesity due to smoking and liver disease
- depression
- Attempts at suicide
- a low level of health-related quality of life
- illegal drug use
- danger of intimate relationship violence
- a number of sexual partners
- STDs (sexually transmitted illnesses)
- Unwanted pregnancies
- fetal demise

Signs of Stress in Children

The indications and symptoms of stress in children differ according to their age. A change in their behavior is an obvious symptom of stress.

When children are under stress, they may withdraw socially. They may quit communicating to friends and relatives or socializing with others. Bedwetting and nightmares are also signs of stress at night. They may also appear to have a loss of appetite or refuse to eat.

Poor performance - as evidenced by worsening grades - or refusal to attend school are "telltale signs of stress."

Furthermore, children who are stressed may acquire harmful coping techniques, so as a parent, you should be aware whether your child is acting out, avoiding something or someone, withdrawing within themselves, or, in extreme circumstances, bullying a peer.

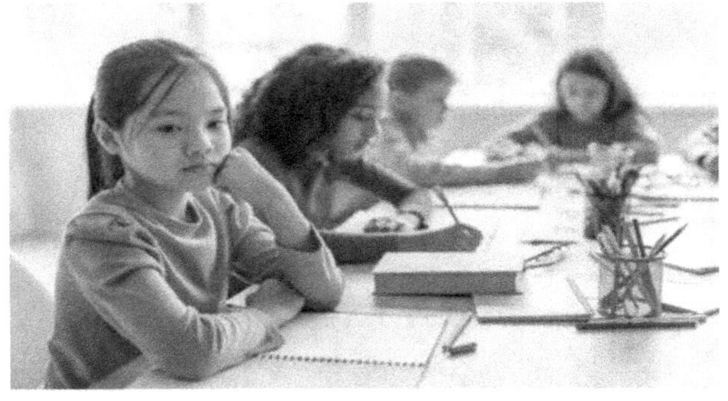

Common Causes of Childhood Stress

To alleviate childhood stress, we must first identify and comprehend its underlying source.

There are three primary sources of stress in children.

- The first are their own and their parents' expectations. They may have low self-esteem or a negative self-perception. Perhaps their parents want them to be top students or force them to do activities they dislike.

- The second factor is peer pressure; kids may feel compelled to comply or do things that their classmates are doing.

- The third factor is family, which can range from difficult parent-child relationships to destroyed homes and abuse.

Helping Your Child Deal with Stress

Children are tough. They can cope with and respond to stress in a healthy manner, but you, as their parents, should provide some assistance and guidance.

What parents can do

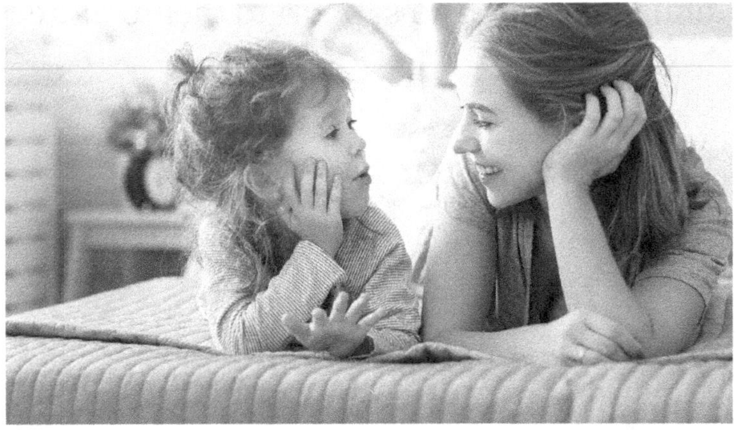

Children must be able to openly communicate with their parents. Make it clear to your child that they can contact you at any moment.

Parents should always speak to their children in a nice manner. Don't merely tell them what to do or how to deal with their situation. You must speak to them gently and inquire as to how they feel and what they are experiencing.

You want your child to be able to communicate with you honestly and safely. Allow them to express themselves. This is not something that happens overnight. It takes some time. So you must be patient. You must communicate to your child that they may talk to and confide in you at any time. Parents must also provide understanding and support to their children.

What teachers can do

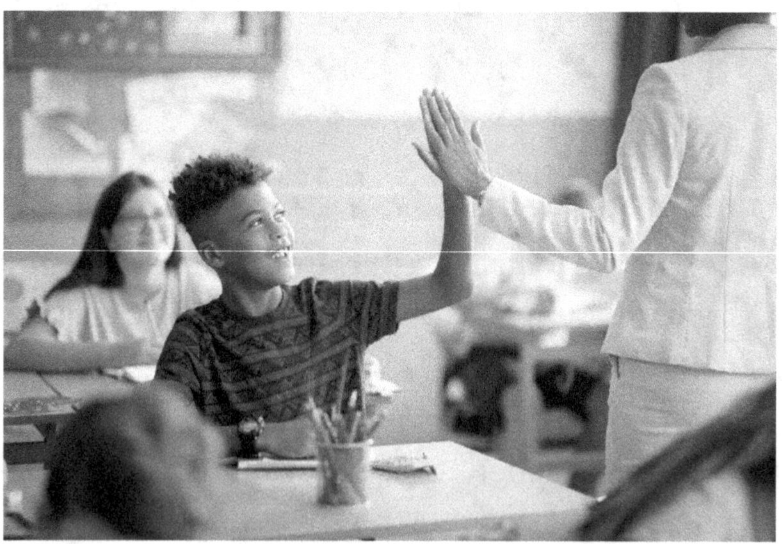

Teachers should monitor children and determine whether or not their students are having difficulty learning.

Teachers can also play an important role in assisting children with stress. A wayward or challenging youngster may be acting out due to stress. Punishing the youngster should not be the initial reaction.

Teachers should be able to watch their students/children and identify any learning abnormalities, such as attention deficit hyperactivity disorder (ADHD) or dyslexia. Don't dismiss the child as being mischievous. Furthermore, he believes that teachers should regard each child as a person with unique requirements.

When should you seek expert assistance?

If the symptoms intensify and begin to interfere with a child's everyday life, he or she may require expert assistance. Dr. Stephen suggests that they speak with school counselors or child psychologists. You might also take them to see a behavioral therapist.

Another alternative is to consult with a family therapist. If your child is having difficulty learning, they may need to consult an educational/learning therapist.

If necessary, the appropriate medical specialists can prescribe medication for attention and focus, anxiety, or depression. In addition, your youngster may benefit from health supplements. You can also create herbal soup for your child to help them relax.

Your youngster can learn healthy strategies to cope with and overcome stress with the right instruction. Parents should also plan their child's daily activities, which should include a decent mix of study, relaxation, fun times, and mindfulness training. According to the American Psychological Association, mindfulness training decreases stress and amygdala reactivity to frightened faces in middle-school children.

Throughout their early years, parents must understand and assist their children. Be the one in whom they may confide. Be their best pal. The youngster can overcome stress and hardships with adequate care and support.

Section 4

Stress-Eating

Understanding Stress-Eating Prevention Strategies

When confronted with a tough situation, the body responds with a 'fight or flight' reaction, defining stress. Stress can help people deal with difficult or dangerous situations. It has an impact on both the mind and the body and comes in two varieties: good and bad. 'Good' stress aids in daily tasks and dealing with obstacles, whereas 'bad' stress can impair a person's ability to deal with those challenges.

Stress, in moderation, can be beneficial; but, when stress levels become difficult to manage, it can have a negative impact on a person's physical and mental well-being. Chronic stress is defined as long-term stress, and it can cause extremely severe symptoms and have a negative impact on an individual. Stress-eating is one of the negative effects of excessive levels of stress.

What is Stress-eating?

Stress-eating is a type of 'binge eating' that occurs when a person is stressed and uses food to make themselves feel better and cope with stress. People that are stressed eat unhealthy, high-calorie items such as chips, ice cream, pizza, and so on. When ingested in excessive quantities over a short period of time, these foods are harmful to one's health.

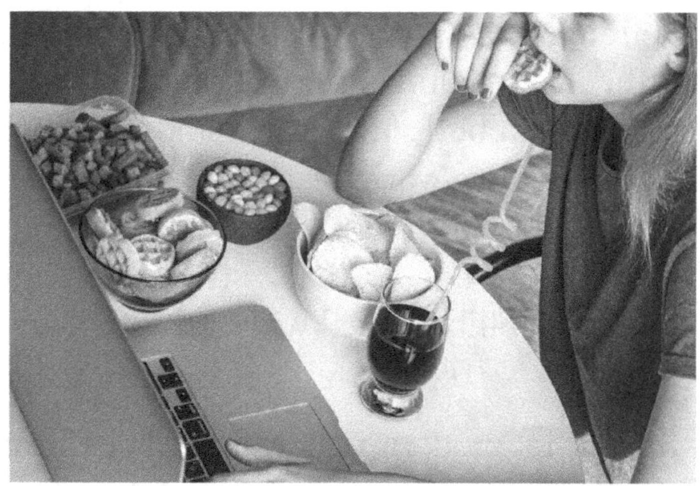

Most people feel disappointed and guilty after eating unhealthy foods, and they begin to feel horrible about their bodies. This causes them even more stress and harms their mental health. This results in an endless circle of tension.

In most situations of stress-eating, the individual increases their food consumption, which can eventually lead to weight gain if it continues for an extended period of time. However, stress-eating can also involve limiting the amount of food ingested, which, if prolonged, can result in weight reduction. Aside from the impacts on mental health, stress-eating can have a negative impact on physical health. Consuming foods heavy in calories, fat, sodium, sugar, and preservatives can increase the risk of type 2 diabetes, high blood pressure, obesity, and other cardiac disorders.

Stress-eating begins as a sort of emotional eating but, if not managed properly, can evolve to a variety of eating disorders such as Binge Eating Disorder (BED) and Bulimia Nervosa.

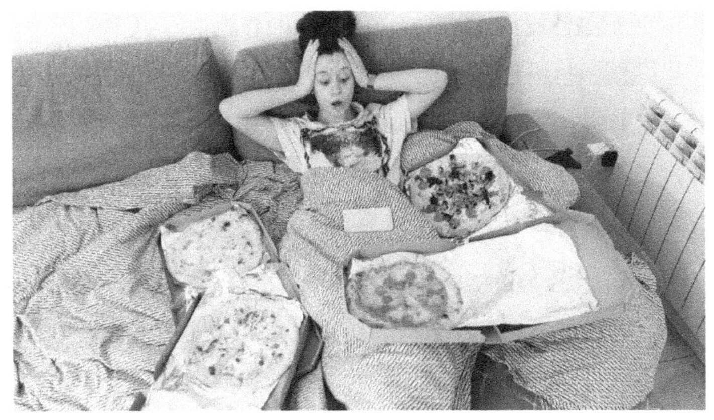

Causes Stress-eating

The following are the primary causes of stress eating:

- **Emotional distress:** Stress-eating is common in those who are experiencing emotional difficulty, such as anxiety, grief, or irritation. Stress can be induced by a variety of circumstances, including illness, the death of a close relative, disagreements, financial difficulties, and so on. Food can provide short relief or distraction from negative feelings.

- **Coping mechanism:** Food is used as a coping method by some people to deal with stress. During difficult times, eating can provide a sense of control and a short mood rise.

- **Habitual Behavior:** Over time, stress-eating can become a learned behavior. If individuals frequently turn to food during stressful situations, it can become a habit.

- **Cravings for Comfort Foods:** Stress may trigger cravings for specific comfort foods that are associated with positive memories or emotional comfort.

How to avoid stress-eating

Recognize the distinction between the urge to stress eat and being hungry.

When people are stressed, they seek specific meals, although hunger can be satisfied by any food. Stress-eating urges must be met immediately and may not be fulfilled even with a full stomach, but hunger vanishes when the person is satisfied. So, before acting on the cravings, the person should be conscious and take 5 minutes to check in with themselves.

Section 5

Foods that will help you relieve stress

Various Healthy Foods, Fruits and Vegetables, Cheese and Eggs.

Green Tea

Many recent researches have shown that Green tea has a calming effect on your body. Given that it is the easiest thing to add to your regular diet, the popularity of green tea has grown in recent days.

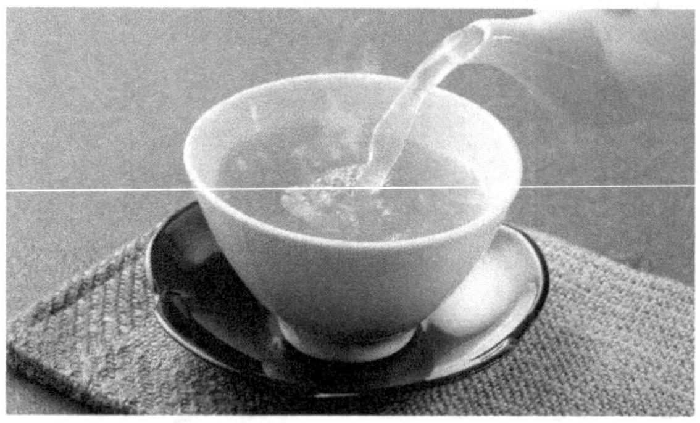

Green tea contains an amino acid called L-Theanine, an amino acid that helps relax the brain. L-theanine is believed to promote brain function by stimulating the production of alpha waves in the brain – relaxing the mind in stressful situations while keeping the brain alert. Studies have also shown that regular drinking of green tea has a positive effect on high blood pressure and high cholesterol.

Yogurt

Yogurt is known as a food that has positive effects on digestion. Recent researches have shown that these positive effects on the digestive tract can also have a positive effect in our brain thereby reducing stress.

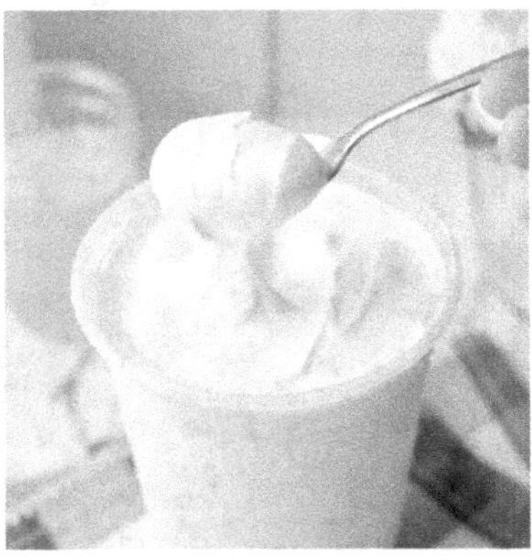

The probiotic bacteria in yogurt was linked with lower levels of activity in areas of the brain responsible for emotion and pain. Due to the healthy management of gut bacteria that directly affects chronic stress, yogurt is recommended as a stress reducing food.

Dark Chocolate

Dark Chocolate has featured in the list of antidepressant foods for a long time. Researchers believe that dark chocolate helps in reducing stress. Researchers believe that the benefit of dark chocolate comes from the rich source of polyphenols, especially flavonoids. Flavonoids help in improving cognitive functions in the brain. Dark chocolate also has high tryptophan content, which the body uses to turn into mood-enhancing neurotransmitters, such as serotonin in the brain. Dark Chocolate is also high in Magnesium. Magnesium relaxes vascular smooth muscle, resulting in vasodilation and increased cerebral blood flow. This helps in improving mood.

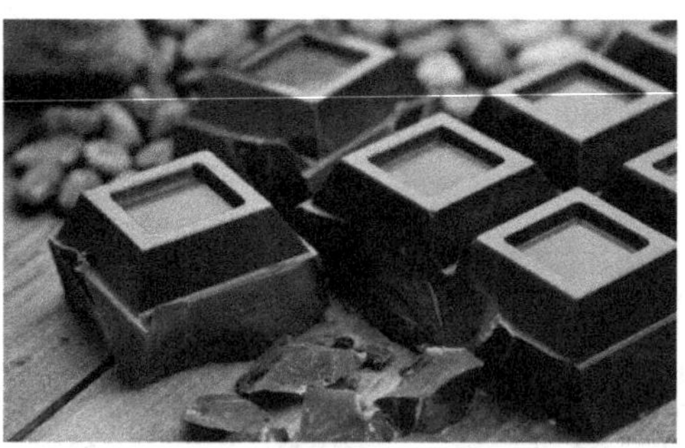

Minerals and Vitamins recommended for Stress Relief

Folic Acid (Folate)

Folic Acid (also known as Folate or Vitamin B9) is a type of Vitamin. Folic acid helps the body produce and maintain new cells. In particular, red blood cell formation is dependent upon adequate levels of this vitamin.

Folic acid has a great role to play in improving the health of your heart and lowering blood pressures. Here is a study that was done to show folic acid improves blood pressure in both men and women. Studies have shown that folic acid has a relaxing effect on the inner walls of the blood vessels. This improves blood flows and thus helps bring down high blood pressure.

In addition, studies have shown that folic acid also prevents you from stroke or heart attacks. Your blood has a type of amino acid known as Homocysteine. You generally get it from eating various foods, especially meat. Homocysteine is known to damage the inner walls of arteries. Such damage can boost the risk of a stroke or heart attack. Folate, along with other B vitamins, helps break down homocysteine and avoid the risk of stroke or heart attack.

How much Folic Acid does your body need? What is better – Diet or Supplement?

When doctors prescribe folic acids, they look at your diagnostic chart, medical conditions and age.

In the majority of conditions 500 mcg to 40 mg of folic acid per day have been used. The greatest benefit seems to occur with folic acid doses of 800 mcg per day or lower. Folic Acid is majorly prescribed by doctors during pregnancy. However, both men and women have a daily requirement of folates. The same can be obtained through food or supplements.

Foods that contain Folate are:

- Legumes

- Leafy green vegetables

- Eggs

- Fruits like Banana, Papaya and Orange
- Vegetables like Beetroot and Broccoli

Natural sources of folic acids are always better. However, there can be conditions where your body is not getting enough folic acid from the foods. In such cases, multivitamin supplements containing Vitamin B9 (Folic Acid) are prescribed.

Do not start taking folic acids just like that. Get your folic acid levels in blood measured and consult a doctor before you start on your supplements.

Iron (Fe)

Iron is an essential mineral in our body. It is an important part of the hemoglobin in blood. Hemoglobin is the protein substance that is present in the red blood cells (RBCs). One important task of red blood cells (RBC) is to carry oxygen from lungs to heart, brain and other parts of the body. Low iron condition leads to decreased levels of hemoglobin in the red blood cells (RBCs). In such a condition RBCs fail to carry the requisite amount of oxygen from lungs to your body tissues. This can result in multiple health problems. While iron deficiency alone may not be the cause of depression, it can lead to similar symptoms as depression like lack of appetite, irritability, extreme fatigue, headaches and mood swings. Research has shown that average ferritin level (a marker of stored iron) was significantly lower in depressed people.

Foods that contain iron are:

- Red meat, pork and poultry
- Seafood
- Beans
- Dark green leafy vegetables, such as spinach
- Dried fruit, such as raisins and apricots
- Iron-fortified cereals, breads and pastas
- Peas

Magnesium

Magnesium is one of the most essential minerals in the human body, connected with brain biochemistry and the fluidity of neuronal membrane. It plays an important role in regulating cortisol levels and prevents excess cortisol production due to its ability to calm the nervous system. A variety of neuromuscular and psychiatric symptoms including different types of depression was observed in magnesium deficiency. There have been reports that over the counter magnesium supplements have helped patients suffering from depression. However, we suggest natural sources of magnesium.

Foods that contain Magnesium are:

- Dark green leafy vegetables, such as spinach
- Almond, Cashew, Peanuts
- Dark Chocolate

Potassium

Low potassium levels have been associated with greater risk for mood disturbances and depression. Potassium appears to act as a facilitator in ensuring the brain's ability to properly utilize serotonin, the neurotransmitter primarily targeted by antidepressants.

Foods that contain Potassium are:

- Dark green vegetables, such as spinach and broccoli
- Potatoes, Pumpkin, Cucumber
- Banana, Orange and Orange Juice

Selenium

There is evidence that uneven selenium status is associated with depressed mood. Research has shown that selenium levels that are both too high in the body, and worse, too low, can place young people at greater risk of depression.

Foods that contain Selenium are:

- Eggs, Chicken, Pork
- Milk, Yogurt and Cottage Cheese
- Bananas

Thiamine

Vitamin B1, also called thiamine or thiamin, is sometimes called an "anti-stress" vitamin because it may strengthen the immune system and improve the body's ability to withstand stressful conditions. Low levels of thiamine are associated with higher risk of depression.

Foods that contain Thiamine are:

- Chicken, Pork, Beef, Fish (Tuna, Trout)
- White Rice, Brown Rice, Whole Wheat Bread
- Orange, Apple

Vitamin D

Multiple researchers have found correlation between depression and low levels of vitamin D. Vitamin D receptors are present in nearly every part of the human body, and so, the ways in which vitamin D might affect your mood are innumerable. One of those mechanisms could be hormonal, since vitamin D helps regulate testosterone levels and low testosterone can impair the mood of men and women.

Foods that contain Vitamin D are:

- Dairy Products (Milk, Yogurt, Cottage Cheese)
- Soya Beans, Soya Milk
- Cod Liver Oil

Vitamin B6

Vitamin B6 helps the body in making several neurotransmitters and chemicals that carry signals from one nerve cell to another. It is needed for normal brain development and function. It also helps the body to make hormones like serotonin and norepinephrine, which influence mood, and melatonin, which helps to regulate the body clock.

Foods that contain Vitamin B6 are:

- Eggs, Chicken, Pork
- Bread, Brown Rice
- Soya Beans, Soya Milk

Vitamin B12

B12 is also involved in the production of serotonin and other neurotransmitters that regulate mood. Due to this, their low levels can cause changes in the nervous system.

Foods that contain Vitamin B6 are:

- Meat, Eggs
- Milk, Cheese
- Cod Liver Oil

Vitamin C

The link between vitamin C and mood might seem surprising, but people who have vitamin C deficiency often feel fatigued or depressed. A deficiency in vitamin C, also called ascorbic acid, can cause neurological damage, and the addition of vitamin C to the diet can improve or reverse the symptoms of anxiety, depression and bipolar disorder.

Foods that contain Vitamin C are:

- Citrus Fruits – Orange, Lime, Lemon
- Red, Yellow and Green Capsicum
- Lychee, Papaya, Banana

Zinc

Zinc participation is essential for all physiological systems, including neural functioning, where it participates in a myriad of cellular processes. Deficiency of zinc leads to diminished functioning of the brain accompanying episodes of major depression.

Foods that contain Zinc are:

- Milk, Yogurt, Cheese

- Peanuts, Cashew, Almonds
- Beef, Lamb, Pork

Omega 3 Fatty Acids

Omega-3 fatty acids are thought to have the most potential to benefit people with mood disorders. Omega-3s can easily travel through the brain cell membrane and interact with mood-related molecules inside the brain. They also have anti-inflammatory actions that may help relieve depression.

Foods that contain Omega 3 Fatty Acids are:

- Flaxseed, Chia Seeds, Walnuts
- Soya Beans, Soya Milk
- Cod Liver Oil, Fish and Fish Oils

Herbal Remedies to Do Away with Stress Effectively

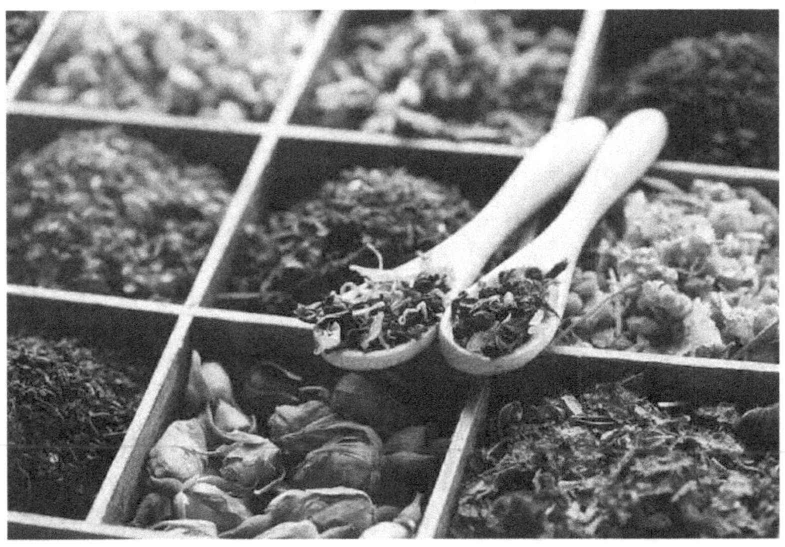

Consuming a herbal formulation that contains flower parts like rosebuds can provide effective stress relief.

Different systems of medicine like psychiatry, Ayurveda and TCM can alleviate stress by helping a person achieve balance. Similarly, the use of traditional herbal remedies can help to promote a better flow of liver *qi*.

- **Rosebuds and mint leaves:** Rosebuds and mint leaves are particularly favorable remedies for stress. The best way to consume these herbals is to soak them in freshly boiled water for approximately 5 minutes before consuming them. Do this 2-3 times weekly. Consuming a rosebuds infusion can also promote increased blood circulation. So, pregnant women or women on their period should avoid using rose petals as a herbal remedy for stress.

- **Lily bulbs and lotus seeds:** Consuming a formulation that uses lily bulbs can help alleviate the symptoms of stress. Lily bulbs consist of three sets of active components: alkaloids, steroidal saponins and phenols. The combination of alkaloids and steroidal saponins, in particular, is responsible for the effective treatment of various nervous system disorders. Lily bulbs are abundant with essential nutrients. Combining it with lotus seeds may treat the symptoms of stress, such as irritability, restlessness, anxiety and insomnia. Before consuming, boil both herbals together for approximately 20-30 minutes.

- **Turmeric:** Curcumin is found primarily in turmeric and linked to multiple health benefits. Turmeric is a medicinal root that contains curcumin, a polyphenol that has demonstrated antioxidant, anti-inflammatory, anti-mutagenic, anti-microbial and anti-cancer activities. The antioxidant and anti-inflammatory activities of curcumin can help improve systemic markers of oxidative stress. At the same time, curcumin can reduce triglyceride — a type of fat — levels and decrease the markers of stress, neurodegeneration, and liver injury in the body. On the other hand, a separate clinical trial found that the use of curcumin was also able to promote calmness and alleviate fatigue caused by psychological stress.

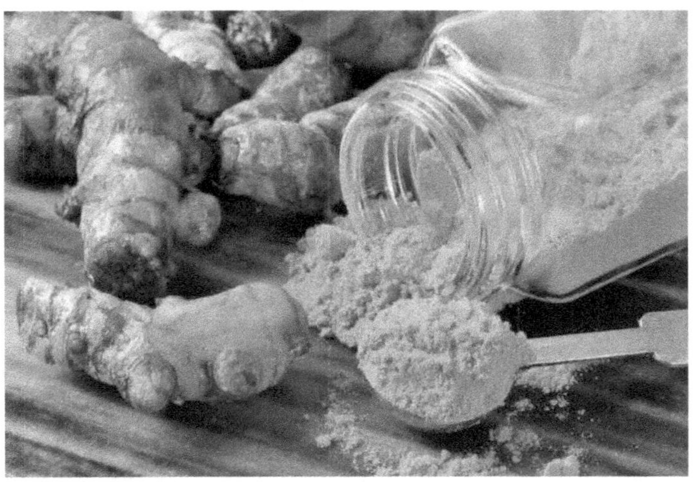

- **Hawthorn berries:** Hawthorn berries in TCM are commonly associated with health benefits. They include decreased cholesterol levels and a reduced risk of cardiovascular disease. It has also demonstrated anti-inflammatory and anti-tumour activities.

Knowing what stress is can help you take the necessary steps to relieve the physical and mental tension. These include the use of natural medicinal remedies, which offer multiple wellness benefits. Do speak to a TCM physician beforehand to ensure that you are choosing the right herbals for you.

Conclusion

In today's high-pressure lifestyle, it is difficult to steer clear of stress completely. Stress is a normal part of life, and some degree of stress can actually be beneficial. However, when stress becomes chronic and overwhelming, it can have negative effects on our physical and mental health. While stress may not be cured or completely eliminated from our lives, many strategies and techniques can be used to manage and reduce stress.

Additionally, it's important to address the root causes of stress, such as work or personal issues, in order to effectively manage and reduce stress in the long term.

And remember, there are not two of you but one. Therefore you should make every effort necessary to do away with anything that will and can stress you out. And never forget that if you should lose your life or your senses from a stressful work or relationship, there shall always be a substitute for you. It should always be you first.

Never lose the sight to the fact that you are the Remedy to stress. Is either you choose to control stress or you let stress control you.

www.ingramcontent.com/pod-product-compliance
Lightning Source LLC
Chambersburg PA
CBHW070728260726
48660CB00007B/2768